Disance Running

for the not very athletic

Don Franks

Copyright © 2018 Don Franks

All rights reserved.

ISBN-13: 978-1717057587

DEDICATION

To the workers who created the Polhill Gully track.

CONTENTS

Acknowledgement	v
Getting started	1
First run	5
Becoming addicted	8
Theory and practice	12
The most difficult time	16
Weighty issues	18
How far, how fast, how frequent?	21
Your first race	25
Gearing up	28
Training and playing	30
Running into trouble	32
The misnamed half	35
Running away	38
The big one	47
A marathon diary entry	51
Epilogue	58

ACKNOWLEDGEMENT

Thanks to Verena Watson for fine-tuning this work.

GETTING STARTED

Distance running makes you feel good and anyone can do it. Documented experience shows that with a few key things in place, all types and ages of people can enjoy running if they want to.

This book is offered as a guide for anyone with fleeting thoughts about getting fitter. It draws from a not very athletic runner's twenty-seven years on the road.

To get underway, you need:

- Time to run
- A place to run
- Running shoes
- A notebook
- Persistence

Time to run

Most of us are busy, many of us too busy. Because it's not renewable, time is the most precious thing we have.

Running demands some time. At first, not much, just three half hours from each hundred and sixty-eight hour week. Three sessions a week is the recognised minimum needed to produce a training effect. If you're very unfit, you will at first just be running a few minutes each session. About the same amount of time we use to brush our teeth each day.

As you grow fitter, running becomes more enjoyable and you'll find yourself devoting more time to it without thinking.

A place to run

Anywhere there's a clear space ahead of you will do to start running. It helps if there's no traffic fumes and a pleasant view. Views can be a handy distraction when early steps demand big efforts. A park, bush trail, beach, waterfront, or playing field is ideal to begin running in. At first, it's best to run somewhere flat.

Running shoes

Sporting and shoe shops stock a bewildering range of running shoes. The only requirement you have at the start is that your new shoes feel comfortable. There's no need to get the most expensive option. Around $150 should be enough to buy an ideal pair that will last you at least a year. Bear in mind that this is the only money you'll need to spend on your new chosen sport.

A notebook

Many beginner runners have found there are good reasons for keeping a diary. Recording the date, length of a run, and any other relevant details, helps make your progress look real.

As you build endurance, it's encouraging to look back and see that what was once quite impossible is now doable, and fun to do.

A running diary keeps you honest, its entries tell you exactly what you have and haven't done. It also acts as a sort of medical record if you note that a run was missed because of some ailment.

Persistence

These days we're used to instant gratification in just about every area of life. Because of the way our bodies work, fitness training takes weeks to produce any noticeable effects. For some of us previously unused to exercising, it's an effort to get out and move initially. It may be uncomfortable, you keep doing it, but nothing seems to be happening. We're all built a bit differently but four or five weeks of regular slow jogging will show definite results. Some of us just have to have faith for a period of time.

You might find it helps to have a running companion. When running with a buddy, you can motivate each other. Team with a friend who's likely to reliably show up.

FIRST RUN

You decide to try the first run of your new training program. Outside of dashes to the bus, this might be the first run you've had in years. Is it really a sensible idea? Might you drop dead from a heart attack? Recollect some of those previous runs for the bus—you survived them without being struck down. A controlled training run is less stressful than an unexpected dash wearing a coat and lugging a bag.

If you haven't been very active lately and are carrying extra weight on your frame, it may be wise to build up with a couple of week's brisk walks. Three walks a week, of about twenty minutes, at faster than your normal walking pace. To be sure of winning a training effect, you should be puffing and sweating a bit at the end of these walks. Your heart, lungs, and muscles will start to get the message that they're going to be used a bit more.

For your first actual run, it helps to walk five or ten minutes beforehand to warm up. Your breathing will then be working better and you'll be less likely to pull a muscle.

The difference between walking and running is not speed. The action of running, however slowly, involves both feet being momentarily off the ground at the same time.

Enjoy the anticipation of your initial run, put on clothes that you feel good in. These will be your nice new running shoes, shorts, a loose fitting T-shirt, and a comfortable bra if required. Pull on a jersey if it's a very cold day but be prepared to shed it because you'll heat up very quickly.

Before taking off, check the time. Don't recheck your watch until you decide you're finished. Your goal at this stage is to run slowly for as long as it feels ok. The time of a first run is different for each individual. In my case, I was unable to complete one whole minute before stopping to gasp for air.

How people feel after unaccustomed exercise varies a lot. If you're absolutely stuffed, don't be discouraged. Dig into your bag of Persistence. If you just stubbornly keep at it, your body will, however grudgingly, eventually fall into line. Future runs *will* go better.

Whatever time you initially make, spend a few extra minutes walking before sitting down. Warm downs are as important as warm ups.

When you get back home, note the date in your diary, with the time spent running. Feel a bit pleased with yourself for getting underway and look forward to your next session. That will be whenever you decide. It may be the next day, whenever. Just as long as you log three sessions a week. Run more times than that in a week if you like, just take at least one day off to recover. If you don't do that your body will become very unhappy and mutinously organise a little injury so that it can rest up a while whether you like it or not.

BECOMING ADDICTED

Your second and third training runs may well be harder than your first go. Human bodies can make all sorts of one-off efforts in emergency situations, but they don't accept emergency as a daily routine.

If you, like me, find the first few runs rather difficult, don't be put off. If you keep at it, you *will* overcome.

Running is dialectical, quantity turns into quality and this change happens quite suddenly. After slogging away dutifully for a while, you'll come to enjoy unexpected days when everything suddenly comes together and you feel you could just go on and on.

Beginning to run is a bit like beginning to smoke tobacco. Unfamiliar, uncomfortable, until you persist, and then you find you're addicted, with each puff doing you damage.

With running, each step is making you stronger. It may help to keep reminding yourself of this fact on days when the last thing you feel like doing is heading out the door in your shorts. The day will come when you find you're hooked, and, if for some reason you can't fit in a run, you get grumpy and twitchy.

When you've finally acquired your full-on running addiction, you just need to keep feeding it.

Some tips for the early, difficult days:

- Don't take peeks at your watch. In this beginner running phase, time will appear to be barely moving, minutes will stretch themselves out to an extent you wouldn't have thought possible.
- Distract your mind with whatever works for you. Thinking through a work project, planning a dinner menu, recalling a cricket game, a movie, or a poem, whatever. In my case, I played tenor horn scales in my head, trying to visualise the valve positions in every key.
- Some runners like listening to music on headphones. I have never tried this and hesitate to recommend it, because you need all your wits about you when running through this world in a T-shirt. Dogs, cars, and cyclists need to be watched out for. You also have to keep an eye on your footing and not trip up. For those sorts of reasons, a park or school playground is an ideal beginner runner's track. You don't have to worry about safety so much and are therefore freer to distract yourself from the struggle of unfamiliar and prolonged movement.
- It pays to consider what surface you're running on. At first, a flat grassy area is the best of all. Because running means both feet being momentarily off the ground, the whole weight of your body smites the surface at every step. The harder the surface, the more your body will be jarred. If you possibly can, avoid running on concrete. tarmac has a little more give in it. Bush trails are better still, with the advantage of being

uneven and therefore using a greater range of muscles. The shoreline of a beach is good, so is an unused golf course. As you continue running, your muscles will develop and your bone density will improve. Along with this, your movement will become more economical and athletic. You'll also lose some weight. In sum, you'll become more adapted to tolerate running on hard surfaces.

- The best time of day to run is what suits your preference. With a full time job or a family to care for, running time is when you can fit it in. Some of us have found running to work manageable, or running home from work. When I was cleaning at Spartan Engineering, it was ideal for me to jog back home because I worked in T-shirt and shorts. My preference now is to run first thing in the morning—it helps me wake up and tune into the day. Morning running is doable for many people because you just need to rise a bit earlier and there's your running time found. If you can time your run for when the dawn is breaking, there's the wonderful feeling of being part of nature's renewal.
- What about if it's raining? Running in the rain actually feels ok if you take a few precautions. A light waterproof jacket is nice if you have one and you definitely need a cap or visor to keep rain from driving into your eyes. If rain comes on half way through a run, I usually find it exhilarating but I hate heading out straight into rain. Instead I'll jog on the spot in the porch for five minutes first; if you're warmed up for it before setting out, rain is more tolerable.

- If it's really cold outside, wear a wooly hat and gardening gloves. That should be enough for most New Zealand winter temperatures.

THEORY AND PRACTICE

"A book! How could there be a whole book just about running!?" a non-running acquaintance said to me. He was considering a half marathon sometime in the future and I'd suggested he borrow one of my favourite running books, of which I have over thirty. As you'll see if you look in the shops, that's only a tiny fraction of the available running literature.

Maybe because our sport is often a solo activity, some runners become introspective and inclined to reflect on and write about their experiences. Whatever the reason, there's thousands of 'How to run' books out there, many of them very good.

As a beginner runner, I found running books inspirational and encouraging. Most of the advice seemed sound, although you'd be surprised how much disagreement there is about the best ways to train and race. If you're doing all your training alone, you may, like me, draw sustaining support from expert runners' books.

It's not necessary to buy running books new. Many of them turn up in second hand shops or are in the public library.

Here, in no particular order, are a few best-selling

running titles that have helped keep me on the road:

Women's Running by Dr Joan Ullyot contains specific advice for women and is also a sound all round title for anyone. It carries the knowledge of a trained medical doctor along with the experience of a keen athlete.

The Runner's Handbook by Bob Glover, a champion runner and professional coach. A substantial work answering many runners' questions, with sensible race training schedules.

The Complete Book of Running by James F. Fixx. The extravagant claim of the title is a product of Fixx's enthusiasm, which tumbles from every page. The author of this famous work is sometimes held up as a reason not to run as Fixx died while running at age 52 (from health issues unrelated to running).

Aerobics by Dr Ken H. Cooper is a pioneering fitness book also applicable to walkers, swimmers, and cyclists. The detailed 'points' accumulating system of gaining fitness will not appeal to everyone, but the science has basically stood the test of time.

Middle Distance Running by Percy W Cerutty dauntingly begins "I hold that suffering and dedication is the only way to understanding … ". Quite a bit of sound advice can be found in the writing of this eccentric Australian coach, whose thinking was before his time in some respects.

Running to the Top by Derek Clayton is another Australian book, by a world record holder. Active in the days before sport had developed into an overpaid profession, Clayton had to balance office work with training all through his career. A role model for would-be runners who are "too busy" to train.

Jogging with Lydiard by Arthur Lydiard with Garth Gilmour. As is well known, Lydiard produced a number of world champion New Zealand runners; his writing reflects the way he drove himself and his students to the limit.

Running and Being by Dr George Sheehan is one of the eight books by this ex US navy doctor. Sheehan's down to earth training advice peppered with eclectic literary quotations irritates some and is treasured by others. He is the author of my favourite comment on the sport:

> "For every runner who tours the world running marathons, there are thousands who run to hear the leaves and listen to the rain, and look to the day when it is suddenly as easy as a bird in flight."

Galloway's Book on Running by top athlete Jeff Galloway is packed with good practical advice. There's an excellent chapter for beginner marathon runners.

Jog, Run, Race by Joe Henderson. The best, I think, of the many similar books churned out by this sports writer, and my favourite single running book of the lot. The marathon training schedule in *Jog, Run, Race* has been criticised for being in too much of a hurry. Most of Henderson's approach I've found to be spot on.

THE MOST DIFFICULT TIME

So you've made a beginning and are now dutifully logging three sessions a week, at something like five to ten minutes each time. If this feels easy and you're happily running much longer than that, don't bother reading this chapter. If your early experience is more like mine and training's a real battle, read on.

According to my running diary of 1991, it was more than a month before I could run longer than eight minutes in one hit. After another fortnight, I recorded "Six times around varsity rugby field, about 15 minutes. Longest run to date, felt like it too!"

From that point, things quite quickly got better for me and half hour runs became routine. Somehow, I'd finally amassed enough fitness for regular slow running to feel normal.

Even if you're not so decrepit as I was, early training days can be discouraging. That's quite normal. Transition from a sedentary to active life demands some effort.

Here are a few tricks that might smooth your way through the critical period:

- Always remember to warm up slowly when you set off. Make it a habit to walk a few minutes first and, when you do break into a run, begin as slowly as you possibly can.

- The way you consciously move yourself can make a big difference. Consider yourself as moving in slow motion, gliding over the ground in a relaxed easy lope.
- Try to keep your shoulders loose and don't clench your fists. Steady, fluid movement is what you're seeking from your legs and arms. Cruising.
- Vary the length of your strides, small flat-footed steps at first and then, stretch out a bit. Experiment to see what stride works best for you.
  - I found the old fashioned notion of counting your blessings helpful in the early days. Be aware that unlike some other people, you have legs, lungs, feet, and other equipment needed to run, in a peaceful environment. It's a good counter to self-pity.

One way or another, just keep to your schedule and somehow keep going through your first weeks as a runner. The good news is that this initial mental and physical adjustment will be the most difficult period of your running career, even if you go on to finish a marathon.

WEIGHTY ISSUES

Soon after escaping tobacco's clutches, I grew unhealthily fat. My first attempts to run were all about seeking weight loss. Not the best reason to start running.

Unless you spend hours and hours at it, the process of running doesn't burn off many calories. However, regular running can help trim your body down, although not in the way you might expect.

As you get into the sport and the exercise becomes part of your life, your eating habits will change. Without giving it a lot of thought, you'll naturally gravitate towards healthier food choices. Vegetables, fresh fruit, and whole grains will become more appealing, heavier fried foods less so. Sure, you may have been eating well before you became active. But if your previous diet was mostly fast food and stodge, your new running body will start demanding some changes.

As you continue running, you'll begin to lose a little weight, mostly because of your altering diet. Up to a point, the lighter you are, the easier it is to run. So you may start questioning whether you really need to eat the amounts that used to seem ok, knowing that any unneeded fat will have to be hauled along the road with you.

Outside of sex, possibly more nonsense has been talked about food than any other subject. Many running books are padded out with diet suggestions and recipes. Lots of runners get into various silly food fads. Competitive racers particularly are often scrabbling round for anything that might cut fractions of a second from their times.

There are no special foods that runners should seek out. The highly competitive Dr George Sheehan said any diet affording him a decent bowel motion before racing would do just fine.

The sane approach to eating has oft been repeated—eat food, mostly plants, not too much. We keep getting sidetracked from that good sense by capitalists working day and night to hook us onto sales of cheap fats and sugars.

If you are carrying a lot of extra weight, you'll enjoy running more by controlling your eating appropriately.

The best guide I've found for this purpose is a little book titled *How I quit overeating and lost 20kg* by Jill Brasell. She argues:

> "You don't have to count calories or grams of fat or use clever diet apps. You most certainly

don't have to starve yourself. All you have to do is decide once and for all to make a PERMANENT change in your eating habits, so that eating "normally" is eating well, not overeating."

The rest of the book explains practical steps towards this goal. One passage relevant to overweight runners:

"Exercise wasn't part of my plan, but one of the first changes I noticed as I began to lose weight was that walking became easier. Lugging my bulk up even gradual slopes used to be an unpleasant effort, but once I got lighter, hills flattened remarkably and I began to enjoy walking again. I'm now inclined to regard exercise as one of the REWARDS of weight loss rather than a way to achieve it."

HOW FAR, HOW FAST, HOW FREQUENT?

Over recent weeks, you've laid a platform and now comfortably manage regular 20–30-minute runs. One famous running writer suggests that you can, if you want, stay permanently at that level and attempt nothing further.

I disagree, for two reasons. If you just stick to slow half-hour jogs three times weekly you'll eventually get bored.

More to the point, it's not actually possible to stay on any level permanently.

Like everything else on the planet, runners are either coming into being or going out of being.

If we live to be very old it's necessary to wind down and go out of being with good grace, but right up until then we must move forward or stagnate. Fortunately the process of moving forward with running is exciting and fun.

There are three main ways we grow as a runner: going further, going faster, and going more frequently.

Each new direction imposes new stress on the body, so it pays not to try them all at the same time.

Going longer

If your usual run is around half an hour, some weekend, or similar freer time, try extending your distance. Do this on a day when you're feeling good, don't have to rush back to work and have the time to rest afterwards.

I found the most pleasurable way to try a longer run was in the bush or by the shore. Beautiful surroundings distract and uplift. I've also enjoyed running round the sidelines of children's Saturday soccer fixtures, picking up on the field game energy.

You may prefer to take your long run with a companion. If you're evenly matched this can work very well, because conversation helps pass the time. (If you're too puffed to sustain an ongoing running conversation, you're going too fast for your present ability.)

Trying to clock up a whole hour is a good test for new runners. Your first hour is very satisfying to record in the diary.

However you go about running longer, remember to drink water before and after. I don't feel a need to drink during runs of up to an hour but we're all different and you might want to carry some along. Or leave it by your jacket while you run circuits of a park.

For longer runs around a New Zealand city, I've found hand basin water in public toilets perfectly ok for drinking.

The day after an unusually long run you might feel like going right out and repeating it. Not a good idea. You need rest to recover. The second or third days after a big run, you may feel a bit stiff in the shins or the hips. These are welcome signs that your body is recovering, getting ready for next time.

Going faster

Running slowly up hills makes good preparation for speed work. Just take it easy going down, because then you're bashing your bodyweight harder against the terrain.

An athletic track is ideal to try speeding up. The surface is custom made and you can time yourself over 440m (once around) or a mile (four times around).

Before doing any sprints, be sure to warm up well first. A slow 440 circuit will be enough; you may, like me, find the first measured 440 never-ending.

To experiment with speed, try a one-minute sprint at the end of your usual half-hour slow run. If you're going as fast as you can, one minute will be heaps.

After that sprint, don't crash to a halt; take another couple of minutes to warm down at a very slow jog.

Going more frequently

There are some keen runners who take pride in "streaking". In this context the term means running (clad) every single day, for months and sometimes years. Runners getting away with this practice are lucky, because human bodies need regular rest from stress.

Running six days a week is a sensible maximum for enjoying the sport without injury. My preference at the moment is no more than three days in a row.

YOUR FIRST RACE

Back in high school, a few kids were really good at running races. Those of us who weren't, tried to avoid participating because we'd just look hopeless.

Fun runs came in some time after the 1960s.

At Hutt Valley High School, instead of fun runs, we had the dreaded 'Bridge Run'. This course, of several kilometers alongside the polluted Hutt River, was compulsory for all third formers on their first school day. Whichever principal originally instituted the Bridge Run knew their business. The seemingly endless, unfamiliar exertion reduced us cheeky twelve-year-olds to a state of compliance.

Long runs were occasional punishment for having dirty physical education gear. A happy thought in my head when leaving high school was that I'd never have to run again in my life.

The silly thing is, virtually all of us once loved running. Before they can properly walk, toddlers will attempt breaking into a run. As they get better balance, running is a favourite thing for pre schoolers to do. A sensation of sheer delight, and one we're able to recapture many years later.

Some lifelong runners never enter a race. Racing

might not be for you either, but I recommend trying it at least once. A race is an adventure. There's a crowd, a contest, an audience, a buzz. That, plus the sensation of being jolted from your comfort zone. You'll probably move faster than your normal lone jogging pace because of being pulled along by the energy of the group. The extra speed will test you and shake you up a bit. If you like huge crowds and a hyped-up atmosphere, you may enjoy a 'Round the Bays' event. If you miss that date, don't worry, there will be a 5k coming soon somewhere near you.

The 5k distance may seem a lot longer that you expected; whether it does or not, you'll get a feeling of what it takes to knock out five kilometers—and later on 10, 21, and maybe even 42.

For now, don't worry about being able to complete the distance. If you're used to jogging half an hour, you'll get through a 5k no trouble.

The 5k event is called a race, but only a very few fit young folks up the front are seriously trying to be first. The rest of us are basically keeping each other company over the distance. There's a fine feeling of solidarity in a fun run. Like any big group of people doing something in common, we reinforce one another in our chosen activity.

To give it a go, just take a look online to see what 5ks are coming up in your region. coolrunning.co.nz will point you in the right direction. As you'll see, there are hundreds of these things going on all over the place. You pay a small entry fee, pick up your number, and show up on the day.

It will help if you rest up and don't drink any alcohol the day before a race. Other than that you need no special preparation. Wear just what you wear for your normal runs, have a big drink of water, and don't eat anything closer than two hours before the start time. Get to the starting line in time to wander round for a few minutes loosening up. If you're normal, you'll be having some nervous feelings, like stage fright. Fears of possible failure. These will evaporate a minute after you get going.

At the start, try consciously to begin slow. The excitement of a race just naturally draws people along; if you begin quicker than your usual pace you may cramp up. Don't worry if the field leaves you behind. As the race unfolds, you'll pass a few people and you will not come in last. (That last runner will be someone who didn't get to read this book!)

As you cross the finish line, bask in the happy feeling of completing a 5k race. Take a drink of water, walk a bit to warm down, and pop on home to celebrate and record the moment in your diary. Daydream about knocking over your first marathon. We'll look at the practicalities of that one soon.

GEARING UP

For your first few five or ten-minute runs, it doesn't matter much what sort of shoes you wear. Once you're regularly running longer, your shoes will start to show wear. Typically, one shoe will fray more than the other, usually on one side of the heel. The more the shoe unevenly wears down, the worse it is for your feet and knees because your leg will not be functioning in proper alignment. Some running books recommend patching your shoes with rubber adhesives. I have tried this and not found it to work. Better ways to prolong the life of your shoes are these:

- Stay off hard surfaces as much as possible. Grass, bush trails, and beaches take less toll of your shoes than roads. They're more pleasant places to run anyway.
- When you buy running shoes, consider buying two pairs. They will not only wear down slower, if you get two different makes they will tax your feet in different ways so you're not using the same muscles in the same way all the time.
- Even the best running shoe will wear out, and at about the same rate as a cheaper one. A regular rotation of cheaper shoes at the rate of one or two pairs a year seems to suit my pocket and my feet.

- Which brands to buy? I was lucky when I bought my first pair of trainers. When I asked the sales guy what was the difference between the middle and very top of the range, he said very little. In his opinion, expensive prices were just marketing ploys.
- My shoe style preference is a heavier model with plenty of cushioning. If you're into speed you'll probably want something lighter. Try a few pairs and trot around the shop in them and go with whatever feels good. Take note, shoe manufacturers keep throwing up new brands all the time and discontinuing perfectly good models. So if you find a kind you really like, get at least a couple of pairs while they're available.

Running shorts of modern synthetic material never seem to wear out. All my shorts came from garage sales several years ago and look like lasting longer than I will.

You may get attached to a particular top. My favourite T-shirt often draws compliments in races. It's red, well-worn, emblazoned "Workers should be running the country".

TRAINING AND PLAYING

Maybe the best thing about distance running is being able to recapture the glorious feeling of being released from school. Off you set, totally free to go anywhere you like, as fast and as far as you like with no one telling you where to go or what to do. I think this sensation can be enjoyed even more if you also program some contrasting, disciplined training into your schedule.

Deliberately working on different muscles will better equip you to run anarchic and free. Every so often, I seek out a place where I can run structured laps undisturbed. An out-of-hours school playground is ideal. After warming up, I'll sprint a circuit, jog one slow, and sprint again. Sometimes I'll follow this by running laps with my arms held above my head, or out to the sides like an aeroplane. Then I'll cover the area skipping from side to side. All these various motions give a more intense workout than ordinary continuous trotting along.

Some folks do training runs holding weights in their hands but this has never appealed to me. Wherever you carry it, the more weight you have on board, the harder you hit the deck, which isn't being kind to your knees or hips. In between laps of the space, I'll stop and stretch my arms and legs. Habitual running tightens up some muscles much more than others, so we need to restore our flexibility. A test is being able to stand and touch your toes. If you can't reach down there easily, you're too tight.

When I'm having a session of running laps, I usually include a few laps jogging backwards. I saw elderly Tai Chi exercisers doing this in Chinese parks years ago. Since then, I incorporate running backwards into my training, finding that I like the sensation. (Also a handy skill for football referees.)

RUNNING INTO TROUBLE

Apparently, there are greater drains on society than boy racers and foreign drivers. Statistics from 2016 show New Zealand's sports injuries cost ACC more than road crashes, with payouts totaling $542 million.

The payment breakdown for sport's toughest top ten goes like this:

1: Rugby Union - $78,242,505

2: Football - $38,295,109

3: Fitness training/gym - $30,552,020

4: Netball - $27,639,333

5: Rugby league - $19,871,754

6: Basketball - $12,896,045

7: Mountain biking - $14,853,034

8: Skiing - $16,461,223

9: Jogging - $8,326,841

10: Snowboarding - $6,533,251

More people go jogging than play rugby, so runners' injuries are comparably much fewer than footy players. Still, we make the top ten of athletes getting sidelined.

With care, your risk of running injury can be greatly reduced.

A major cause of our injuries is enthusiasm. Once we get the running bug, many of us start training too hard and too fast. Our bodies don't like this and protest. Bits of our carcass suddenly take direct action to get us off the road for a while.

Seventeen years ago, I suffered a typical overly keen runner's injury. At the time I was working as a university cleaner and in training for a marathon, which was five months away. Eager to do a respectable time, I increased my training amount to almost double.

All was going well I thought, until early one morning on the cleaning job I felt pain in both knees. Next morning the pain was worse. Suddenly, I was shuffling round, sore, unable to keep up the rapid pace needed to complete my cleaning round in time. The pain was becoming dreadful and I could hardly walk at all.

Fortunately, I had an idea where to turn. Several of my running books argued that most knee pain comes from the feet and the best remedy is seeing a podiatrist, preferably a podiatrist who's also a runner.

Dr Tim Halpine is one of those guys. He got me to walk across the room, said "Hmmmm", and straight away made plaster casts of my feet. These were blueprints for custom made orthotics, which cost ACC $400.

"Wear these all the time, don't run for a fortnight, and then ease back into it."

I did what Dr Tim said and, five months later, ran the full course of my marathon.

A good podiatrist is the runner's best friend. We all have some imbalance in our feet, overtraining will highlight this and pass the problem along to our bodies weakest link, the knee. Well-made orthotics bring our balance back into line.

Experience suggests that we should increase training slowly. Try and do most running on grass, beaches, or trails. Always warm up and warm down. Take at least one rest day a week and several days off after a long hard race. It's better not to go out running if you're feeling hung-over or very tired, because you'll be less likely to pick up your feet properly and be more inclined to trip over. That formula won't prevent all possible running injuries. Just most of them.

THE MISNAMED HALF

Longer road races can totally be doable (and fun) for the not very athletic. All we need is to prepare and pace ourselves properly.

For my money, the best race distance of the lot's the half marathon. Long enough to be a memorable adventure, but not so tough that it knocks you out for weeks.

I just wish this classic distance had a more appealing name. There's nothing 'half' about running for over thirteen miles. That's once and a bit right around Wellington's Miramar Peninsula, a fair way to travel on foot.

In terms of time, half marathons take an average 30–40–50-year-old beginner runner roughly two to two and a half hours. It may take you more, that doesn't matter. Your goal is simply to finish.

The key to enjoying a half and finishing it without too much grief is doing a habitual weekly long run some months beforehand. Once a week, make one of your runs substantially further than your norm. You might like to make your pace slower than usual, but the main thing is finding your own natural cruising speed. After you've warmed up and got a second wind you will, on a good day, settle on a natural rhythm. Once you've had the feel of an easy lope along, you'll be able to find that body setting again, and be able to pull it out on race day.

Some say it's best to run the whole distance sometime before racing it. If you can manage that, fine, but I don't think it's essential. If you regularly include an hour's run each week and have once or twice clocked ninety minutes, you're good to go with a half.

At least a week before race day, reduce your training. You can't get any fitter by running longer just before the race. What you need at this stage is energy conservation. The week before race day, do no more than three 20–30-minute runs. The day before, do nothing,

There's no need to carbo load for a half marathon, just eat what you normally have, and take no alcohol the day before.

Check that your toenails don't need trimming. Over a big distance, long nails can cause trouble.

Most half marathons begin mid-morning, at 10 or 11. If you can swing it, arrange to have the afternoon and evening off, because you'll either want to celebrate or just crash out and rest.

As with any long distance race, start slow, and warm up naturally, in whatever time that takes you.

There will be water stations along the way, staffed by kind volunteers. Whether or not you're feeling thirsty, take a drink of water at each station. If it's a very hot day, take two cups each time; drink one and pour the other one over your head.

Sometimes talking with other runners will help keep you going. A distance race is a big party where running lubricates instead of alcohol. Runners of similar pace can and do fall into conversation with each other about all kinds of things.

Should you feel tired at any stage of the race, slow to a walk. Walking for a few minutes can be a good reviver. Stop and stand still for a minute if you need to but sitting down does not help at all, it tells your body that the job is over. Don't sit down unless you've decided to drop out. Pulling out of a race is sensible if you're feeling very unwell. If you've trained properly though, you should be able to find the finish line.

It does not matter in the slightest how long you take to finish. A very slow time just means it will be easier to clock your personal best in the next race.

RUNNING AWAY

If you're lucky enough to afford some overseas travel, running can enhance your visits. Trotting round early morning back streets, you get a close feel of a foreign country. Some of its less familiar sights and sounds and smells.

For example, some diary entries from my trips ...

United States

On my first morning in California, I had a run. In the drizzle, Berkeley looked grainy and bleak. It was, after all, the middle of winter. Tough looking black crows cawing above traffic noise made the soundtrack.

In one direction was a wet concrete shopping area, 7/11, Jack in the Box, liquor stores, and several places advertising Nails. Not hardware nails, manicure. Down the next street were rug and textile shops from Pakistan and Nepal, Wells Fargo bank, Op shops, bars, garages, several vets. A couple of vet places were already open, for dog owners. In America I saw one single cat. In Berkeley the style is dogs, mostly big, much loved, almost everywhere. I began to wonder if dog ownership was compulsory.

Trotting back the other way I passed residential streets, leafier, mostly stucco bungalows, nice, slightly Spanish looking with cacti. Hardly any homes had front fences; apparently, most houses have alarms you need to turn off when coming home.

Back to the 7/11 for a chilli dog, by this time the beggars had clocked on. Showing more style than Wellington beggars. It felt like they were doing you a favour. Each with a confident "spare a few cents to get me a hot meal?" or "Man, you got some change so I can get the bus across town this morning?" Rummaging for the first guy, I found only about twenty cents in my pocket. "That's ok brother, that's ok," said my client in forgiving tones. "God bless you brother. You looking good, I really love your sweater, you have a great day now." Guiltily compensating, I handed the next hustler a note, thinking it was a dollar. It was actually rather more. Oh well. Stuck waiting together for the crossing lights to change, my new friend felt obliged to offer value for the windfall. "God bless you sir. I really love your accent. You're a good man. You know what sir? I can so easily tell you're a Capricorn. No? Ok, of course, I know, you got to be a Leo … ". The Virgo and the beggar were saved by the lights.

By the end of my stay I just about knew each appellant by name. There are a lot of homeless in Berkeley and Oakland, clustered in rope and plastic encampments of several people. Most of them have their bedding in a trolley or pram, many of them have a dog. Like the other citizens, a vehicle and a dog, just in down-market versions.

Cuba

If you want to take a dawn run around old Havana's back streets, you really have to watch yourself. Not for fear of being mugged, but because the pavements are so wrecked. Cracks and deep holes, in some places hastily patched with cement. Various rubbish lies around many of the streets, dog shit, bottles, cans, piles of foul smelling plastic bags. Early morning is when feral cats emerge, clawing rubbish bags to find their breakfast.

In the old section of town there are few public litter bins. Jumbo-sized, four-wheel plastic bins are all over the place, but with seemingly no efficient system of servicing these. At one corner, a little old guy was slowly sorting a vast rubbish heap to separate cans and glass into oil drums. Some of the mess may be residue from recent hurricane street flooding but I guess probably not all.

Outside the shops, it was tidier; several people were out carefully sweeping frontages. In this context, "shops" means one small room with a counter open to the street. Behind the wooden counter will be bottled water, soft drink, cigarettes, beer, and rum. A few of these slots offer cookies or pizza to early morning commuters. It's hard to tell these shops from private homes, because the shops have no signage and Havana homes are not private. At many hours of the day and night, household doors and windows stand open or ajar. Less than a yard from the footpath a householder is visible, mopping a floor, or serving a meal, a family sits watching television, children sort their stuff out for school. The interior furniture tends to solid antique carved wood, paper and plastic flowers proliferate, some large religious icons hang on walls. As the day wears on, older folks come and settle on their doorsteps to socialise. Sometimes playing chess, often puffing big cigars, occasionally sharing rum. Before dawn though the streets are fairly empty apart from taxi cabs and silent groups of workers waiting by bus stops.

I found my way down to the seawall where a few blokes were fishing for spotties. At the shore, a little dog attached itself to me. I crossed the road a couple of times and retraced my steps but the thing kept trotting at my heel until I cut back into a particularly malodorous alley and the dog declined to follow. It was a cute wee mutt but Foxy would not have been impressed if I'd brought it back to Holloway Road.

As the new day got lighter, the streets were suddenly

brightened by the entrance of school children. Chattering and jostling along, the littlest ones hand-in-hand with a parent, each of them wearing a spotless uniform. Ironed white shirts, boys in brown or maroon pants, girls with the same coloured skirts. The youngest kids wore silky blue or red neckerchiefs. Everywhere we went in Cuba the school kids were turned out like this.

Our homestay in Trinidad was on the outskirts of town, bordering farmland. On the first morning there, I trotted down a rutted dirt road past stables and pigsties. As the road narrowed, dogs barked more aggressively and the houses got smaller, some little more than homemade shanties. From these rough dwellings, in ones and twos, came the local schoolchildren, all as neat and scrubbed as their urban cousins. Travelling across Cuba I saw a great many children of all shapes and sizes, not a single one not looking healthy and cared for.

Ireland

A delayed flight from Heathrow plus an airline losing my suitcase delayed my entry to the Dublin hotel until a few hot sweaty minutes short of midnight. Arrival time should have been around 5pm, complete with luggage. Now, my carry-on bag would have to suffice for two days. Spare socks, running shorts, razor, and

Jane Austen makes an almost perfect survival kit. The bed was much comfier than home too, but who's going to sleep first night in the Emerald Isle?

Around 4 o'clock I gave up the effort, brewed tea at the mini bar, used the razor and headed down town.

Cold air blew from the river, workers cycled over the bridge, a keg delivery rattled by the nearest pub.
Down along the riverside, I trotted my three miles an hour, stopping where a couple of neatly geared young guys loitered
"What's the name of the river mate?"
"Ah, this is the Liffey. Out having a run to clear your head then?"
"Sort of."
The shorter guy grinned, twirling a glass of wine in his fingers. "We've not been to bed yet."
"You don't want to be swimming here," cautioned the other bloke. "The water's full of shit."

Taking the advice I headed on over the bridge. On the other side, I got flagged down by a middle-aged Indian couple in a car. "Could you please tell us which is the right way to the airport?" Spaced-out in irresponsible holiday mode, I was still able to resist the temptation to invent long directions in an Irish accent. My honesty was rewarded a few yards later on with a little windfall. A brand new Ed Sheeran concert T-shirt, my size, discarded on the footpath.

Not a huge fan, but something to wear until the airline located my frigging suitcase.

China

Returning there after forty years, I again felt at home in China, but this time round I would not be happy to stay there. Not because of being a frustrated socialist, because of being a runner. Runners, even very slow ones like me, breath air in deep. After two days in China this time, I developed a cough and occasional headaches, which I normally never get.

China's air pollution is constant and severe. Some days the sun is all but blotted out by khaki-coloured smog. It wasn't like that back in the seventies. If I shut my eyes, I can recall a scene, clear as a photograph. The front yard of a PLA military base, a massive lychee tree, all framed by bright blue sky. Now, only on some days, after heavy rain, can blue sky be seen over China.

The pay-off for this industrial pollution is pretty massive. Mile after mile of vast flyovers snake above and around the cities. Thousands of new apartment blocks tower in clusters everywhere. Huge flash hotels have sprung up all over the place, each one we stayed in could have easily fitted our house and section inside the front lobby.

The vast airport and railway station buildings rise so high that you can hardly make out the ceilings. The high-speed passenger trains run smoothly past paddy fields at up to 300k per hour.

Then there's all the billions of clothes, shoes, watches, appliances, tools, kitchenware, textiles, food items, musical instruments, and other stuff produced in China, for home consumption or overflowing to the rest of us. The baby grand I played at the wedding gig was one of around 450,000 pianos made in China every year.

For all that, the pollution is pretty bad and needs fixing. It's not as if Chinese people don't care about their environment. In many respects they are almost obsessively clean and green. Everywhere you travel, street sweepers carefully scoop up every last little bit of rubbish and litter. Mile after mile, the sides of railway tracks are lined with carefully trimmed hedges and bushes. Most trees have the bottom yard of their trunks painted white, to reflect away light and conserve moisture. Any tree on a bit of a lean gets to be carefully propped up by bamboo framing.

On the last morning of our stay in Wuhan, I went for an early run. Out of the hotel grounds, down the side of the main highway. The hotel was out in a light industrial area, miles from any shops or city centre.

Along one side of the misty highway I went, beside the sculpted shrubs, and leafy trees. After half an hour I saw a figure on the other side of the four lane. An older woman in a big straw hat, sweeping the sidewalk with a broom of branches. In slow steady motions, she swept up fallen leaves. The road stretched away before her, as far as her eye could possibly see was

leaf-strewn walkway. I wondered how far she was required to sweep. If her head was locked into some sort of Zen sweeping trip or just counting the bloody minutes until the shift ended.

Then I realised that on my identically treed side of the road, there were no leaves. Someone had swept them

all up before I came out to run. The lady kept sweeping and I kept running. I got tired first and headed back home.

I won't be around to see it, but I'm confident that the Chinese people will someday, somehow, get it together and sweep away their pollution.

THE BIG ONE

"If you want to run, run a mile. If you want to experience a different life, run a marathon."

Olympic champion Emil Zátopek was right. And you don't have to be an Olympic medalist to share the marathon experience. You don't even have to be very athletic. Proof of that is I've done one myself.

There's a fascination with the marathon. What makes the famous distance special is the last six of its twenty-six miles, three hundred and eighty-five yards.

Experimentation and research have confirmed fairly conclusively that normal human bodies aren't meant to run more than twenty miles in one go. After twenty miles, we've used up all our store of glycogen, the glucose energy storage in humans and other animals. When there's no more glucose, our body will reluctantly start drawing on its precious store of fat. It's much easier for us to burn glycogen than fat; out of glycogen, we run less efficiently.

At the same time, after twenty miles, our legs are feeling like concrete. Our hips, thighs, shins, and feet hurt. In solidarity with the rest of the body, our brain starts bombarding us with messages to stop moving. At this stage, the only organ still on our side is our guts.

The marathon is tough but willpower can get us over the line. If we've carefully made the right preparations.

To finish a marathon you need to have at least two years of regular running under your belt, preferably more. You should be taking a long run each week, "long" being more than an hour. You should have completed several half marathons without too much trouble.

All the advice for the half marathon is applicable, except it goes double. For the double distance, you also need some extras.

For those who like specific training schedules, there are many on offer, online and in the running books previously suggested in this book. Compare a few, see what suits you best, and adapt to fit your preference.

I think the most essential thing is taking at least a couple of three-hour runs during your months of build up. These will condition your body to the feel of a very long run. They will also give you the feel of completing a definite running assignment, even if the last part of it is uncomfortable. Don't forget to taper right off in the pre race fortnight. You will not lose fitness and at this stage what you need most is rest.

To keep yourself upright over twenty-six miles, your "core"—stomach muscles—must be strong. Sit-up types of exercise every day will help a lot.

It would not help to carry a ten kg bag of spuds around the course, but you may have the equivalent hanging in places on your person. People markedly overweight for their height handicap themselves for long races, so without making a fetish of it, try to keep your weight in balance.

A first marathon for an average older person will take anything between four and six hours. If your time for the half was two hours, you won't do the full course in four. Set a goal time if you like, but your real mission is to finish.

There are many marathon courses around New Zealand. Not all of them are dead flat, which is what you want on your first outing. Consider the nature of the course—is it out and back, two or three loops, or one long line? Your previous racing experience may have given you a preference. Shop around and choose your preferred course, also your preferred time of year.

Once you're on the road and underway, your feet and legs have struggles ahead. That's nothing remotely approaching the struggle that will take place in your head. After all your pre race preparation, the actual marathon running is mostly mental. A battle between Common Sense (which wants you to give up) and Stubborn Will (which is, today, your true friend).

Suitable bedtime reading the night before race day is John Bunyan's *Pilgrim's Progress*.

After crossing the finish line you'll be completely stuffed. Don't flop down straight away, walk round a few minutes even if you feel like a zombie. You need that movement to settle your body down and get the blood flowing easy. An hour or so later, you'll likely not be able to walk at all. If you can, take a long hot bath and don't do any running for a few days, even if you want to.

All sounds pretty grim, doesn't it? There is a pay-off: crossing the marathon finish line means you've just conquered the universe, as any marathoner will confirm.

A MARATHON DIARY ENTRY

I wrote this account in January, 2001, two days after completing the race. My intention was to try and record, as accurately as possible, what the experience was like. I knew that the longer I waited after the marathon, the more likely it would be for my brain to rearrange, 'with advantages', what had actually taken place. For that reason, I have not edited this little report at all since initially setting it down.

Dark windy Sunday morning.

Grey suburb of Kilbirnie dead and deserted except for the all-night service station.

Buy a Sunday paper and head through the evil looking gloom towards St Pat's College race headquarters.

Under a dim light two volunteer race officials wait at a table, ready to help.

"Come to pick up your number?"

"Got it yesterday thanks."

Nothing to do now but sit and digest the muesli bar and banana shake forced down at five a.m.

Other runners drift in by ones and twos. All look lean and fit and hungry; maybe the next one will look softer or fatter than me?

No chance. Next is a young Asian bloke, all firm, smooth muscle, encased in a silky red singlet. Probably an international star who came all the way to New Zealand just for this race.

He's followed in by another young guy wearing a peaked hanky on his head. Another whippet. Surely there's some other plodders entering besides me.

Never mind that. Just sit in the hall reading the Sunday paper as a distraction from worrying about the run. Nothing can be done to improve chances by worrying now.

"But you are quite a bit undertrained according to most of the books. Wouldn't it be embarrassing if you couldn't hack it and had to pull out before finishing?"

Shut up and read the bloody paper.

Lurid article about the Gary Glitter pornography trial, just what the doctor ordered; able to forget about the race for several minutes.

The forecasted rain has yet to come, but wind keeps on bashing around outside the hall.

"Worst day we've had for it for years," grumbles one of the race officials to his mate. But none of the lean fit hungry looking runners look downcast about it. That lot are perpetually bright and cheery, whatever the weather. They must fly them in from some other planet.

Time to go. We head out onto the road, get a few directions and:

We're off!

Right on cue, the regular pre half marathon feeling bubbles up. *"Really, this whole thing's a bit ridiculous— we've got over thirteen miles to go and all we're doing is a few little shuffling steps. How can we possibly make it all the way? And this time there's not just thirteen plus, there's ..."*

Shut up, and remember the advice about starting. One of the few things all the running writers agree on is you should hold back a bit at the start, especially the start of your first marathon.

Concentrate on holding back until the rest of the field is out of sight. That's ok. You're supposed to run your own race and not be bothered about keeping up with the Joneses.

Despite that, breath is short after less than a mile.

Time to relearn the difference between solo runs and racing.

Races apply their own special pressure.

Even if you struggle to keep slow you're always dragged along faster than usual by the race occasion.

So, along we're dragged, down the road to the coast and round the grass traffic island at the end of Sutherland Road. Glance back to discover one or two actually running behind.

Encouraged by this totally unexpected ego boost, cruise happily along Lyall Bay towards the airport.

The start of Moa Point Road beside the airport includes a complimentary tail wind. Watch it! Don't get carried away in the first eighth of the run!

Round the corner to the first drink stop. Decided last night to walk the length of each water station drinking a full cup. Water and cheering words from friends at the drink stop help the next few bays glide past quite nicely. Up the Pass of Branda and down through Seatoun to the Marine Parade.

There's the first quarter done, in just on an hour, but can't maintain that on my amount of training.

Horrid thoughts of humiliating capitulation start crawling into the head. *"You might not be able to make it …"*

Hold it right there!

You know you can jog at least three hours, so just do that and then walk all the rest if that's what it takes.

The weather's holding up so far. Enjoy the harbour views.

Past the cute little houses around Karaka Bay. Recall that on the first half marathon it started to get hard around here. But that was eleven halves ago, and it's not a problem today.

Exchange a few words with another runner. She's done nine of these before and her goal this time is to finish, running all the way. Looks like she'll have no problem. Pass her to keep up natural cruising pace, but get overtaken again when walking through the next water stop.

Round the scraggly woods of Mahanga Bay. Double boost at Point Halswell. It's the last leg of the first lap and there's a back wind all the way. If that's still there next time round, it will blow us all safely home.

Finally reach Kilbirnie Park. Halfway mark. Involuntary stock take.

"You're hot and tired and your hips are starting to ache, and now on top of that you've got to do it all over again … "

Hey, come on! Cut that out. Look at it this way—half the course done in just over two hours, surely you can repeat it, somehow. Even if it takes six hours. Even if you walk every step. You can do anything you like except pack it in, ok? Ok?? Ok.

First short walk alongside the airport, plus stop to retie laces (no problem with shoes or any other equipment). Keep chugging round to Pass of Branda and walk all the way up it. Welcome slope down to the shore, past a slow sedate runner who's all wrapped up in a tracksuit and there's three quarters of the course done!

Now you know you can do it!

"But I might suddenly feel too stuffed to even walk."

Bullshit. You could walk for the rest of the day if you had to. Walking feels like nothing after running. It feels nice to do.

Have another little walk now.

Increasingly harder to resume jogging after walks. That doesn't matter. Finishing is going to happen, and could even be under five hours. Keep jogging and catch up to a shagged out looking walker. He looks a bit familiar ...

It's the bloke in the red singlet! Shuffle past him and creak on round to Point Gordon, ready to walk the next two bays. At the point who should be walking but the young guy with the hanky hat!

He's a German visitor who's done about ten marathons, but couldn't train properly for this one because of travelling. We walk together for a bit.

"I usually do three hours, but this will be five," he complains.

Five will do me.

Round Point Halswell and get another reviver. The sight of the finish line across the bay and the wind behind combine to produce magic.

Enough magic to resume jogging. Jog like a glacier on valium all the way to Cobham Drive.

Reach the last drink station feeling cheeky.

"Are there any runners in front of me mate?"

"Just a few," says the volunteer giving me the water.

I'll make it under five hours now even if the sky falls in.

Walk half of Cobham Drive and break into a trot at the sign that says 1KM TO GO. Going to make it!! Feel like weeping with relief. Instead, just keep clumping along at half a mile an hour with a silly grin all over my face.

Two kids pop up out of nowhere. One sings out sarcastically:

"Keep going—you're going to win!"

That kid may never be more right about anything in his life.

(My official finishing time: 4 hours 38 minutes.)

EPILOGUE

Mid-morning it was back then, mid-morning in midsummer, the day getting hot and no clouds above the valley.

I took a long break from chopping willows and sat gazing across the Jerusalem Pa. No one was about outside and no cars were on the road, yet I gradually got a deep-seated feeling of things moving.

The old brown Whanganui River down across the road moving, although it didn't look it. Fresh sap weeping from the chopped branches. Atoms in the steel axe head and its wooden handle. Molecules in the air. The feel of everything moving, including me, sitting still but with blood pumping, my body's atoms all charging around.

Everything moving and everything changing. The river never in one spot for a second, the end of my cigarette burning away, myself getting older with each fleeting second. A feeling of things moving and changing. With this, a profound feeling of connection.

A year or so later, reading Engels's *Dialectics of Nature*, I was reminded of my moving/changing feeling back at the commune. This guy was writing, with more elegance and depth, about exactly the same stuff.

Several years after that, when I began distance running, I was reminded again.

Settling into a long easy run reminds the brain that we're matter, in motion, in a constant state of change. Running systematically puts our individual state of change into a positive setting of change for the better. New networks of blood vessels developing, our lungs, heart, muscles, and our mental determination all growing stronger.

More importantly than that to me is that when running, I feel connected to the rest of the constantly moving universe. A feeling of somehow playing an appropriate part, a feeling of belonging.

Running long distances connects the body and calms the mind. Often I've set out for a run unhappy about something; always the unhappiness is diminished, if not completely blown away. I have never returned from a run feeling worse than when I began.

The "runner's high" is a real sensation, although it can't just be summoned up at will. It will come on occasion, unexpected, on days when you are running easily and well—in my case, around forty or fifty minutes into the journey. The high is, well, a high. At least the equal to any sensation I've had from dope, acid, or alcohol.

Like any kind of happiness, the good things coming from running are a by-product. In a universe where everything changes and moves, humans sometimes get out of kilter, because we don't move enough and we have illusions that some things stay the same.

When we run as little toddlers, we're connected up to the cosmos. If we return to running in later life, at any age, we're able to reconnect.

ABOUT THE AUTHOR

Don Franks is a socialist distance runner drawn to the piano.
He has authored *Hill Run*, *Next to Gods*, and *Nice Work If You Can Get It*.

Made in the USA
San Bernardino, CA
24 May 2018